The Keto Chaffle Cookbook

Delicious Savoury and Sweet Low Carb Chaffles that Boost Your Metabolism, Keep You in Ketosis and Make Your Fat Loss Journey Effortless

© Copyright 2019 – Michael Zollo, All rights reserved.

The content contained within this book may not be reproduced, duplicated or transmitted without direct written permission from the author or the publisher.

Under no circumstances will any blame or legal responsibility be held against the publisher, or author, for any damages, reparation, or monetary loss due to the information contained within this book, either directly or indirectly.

Legal Notice:
This book is copyright protected. It is only for personal use. You cannot amend, distribute, sell, use, quote or paraphrase any part, or the content within this book, without the consent of the author or publisher.

Disclaimer Notice:
Please note the information contained within this document is for educational and entertainment purposes only. All effort has been executed to present accurate, up to date, reliable, complete information. No warranties of any kind are declared or implied. Readers acknowledge that the author is not engaging in the rendering of legal, financial, medical or professional advice. The content within this book has been derived from various sources. Please consult a licensed professional before attempting any techniques outlined in this book.

By reading this document, the reader agrees that under no circumstances is the author responsible for any losses, direct or indirect, that are incurred as a result of the use of information contained within this document, including, but not limited to, errors, omissions, or inaccuracies.

Table of Contents

Introduction 2
   Points to Remember to Make Perfect Chaffles 4

Chapter 1: Basic Chaffle Recipes 5
   Basic Keto Chaffle with Egg and Mozzarella 5
   Basic Keto Chaffle with Egg, Mozzarella and Almond Flour 7
   White Bread Keto Chaffle 8
   Rye "Bread" Chaffle 9
   Vegan Keto Chaffle 10

Chapter 2: Breakfast Sweet Chaffle Recipes 11
   Chocolate Chip Chaffle with Whipped Cream 11
   Cream Cheese Chaffles 13
   Chocolate Chaffle 15
   Banana Chaffle 16

Chapter 3: Savory Breakfast Chaffle Recipes 17
   Avocado Toast 17
   Scrambled Egg Chaffle 19
   Keto Cornbread Chaffle 21
   Garlic Parmesan Chaffles 22
   Bacon, Lettuce and Tomato Breakfast Sandwich 23

Chapter 4: Lunch Chaffle Recipes 25
   Bruschetta Chaffle 25
   Spread the topping over the chaffles. Drizzle oil on top and serve. Italian Chaffle Sandwich 26
   Reuben Chandwich 28
   Ranch Slaw Sandwiches 30
   Pulled Pork Sandwich 32
   Tuna Salad Chaffle Sandwich 34

Chapter 5: Dinner Chaffle Recipes 36
Corndog Chaffle 36
Keto Sausage Ball Chaffle..37
Chicken Sandwich 38
BBQ Chicken Chaffle 40
Keto Taco Chaffle 41
Place taco meat in the taco shells and serve with suggested toppings. Chaffle Pizza...42

Chapter 6: Vegan Chaffle Recipes 45
Savory Chaffle 45
Churros Chaffle 46
Chocolate Chaffle 47
Vanilla Belgian Chaffle 48
Pumpkin Chaffle 50

Chapter 7: Snack Chaffle Recipes 51
Chaffle Churro 51
Breadsticks..52
Pickle Flavored Chaffle Sticks 53
Garlic Breadsticks 54
Savory Cauliflower Chaffle Sticks...56

Chapter 8: Dessert Chaffle Recipes 57
Blueberry Chaffle Muffin 57
Nutty Bread Pudding 59
Ice Cream Chaffle Sandwich 61
Strawberry Shortcake Bowls 63
"Apple" Fritter Chaffles 65
Sugar Cookie 67

Conclusion 69
References 71

Free Report , The 7 Keto foods you need to avoid

As a thank you for choosing my book I'd like to offer you a free report I have which talks about the 7 Keto Foods you need to avoid in order to make this journey as healthy and as successful as possible

On top of this I will tell you about the 4 popular diet tips you should NEVER follow. Simply go to www.vipketoreport.com and join my VIP community and I will send it to you instantly, it won't cost you a dime.

To download your copy, go to

www.vipketoreport.com

Any questions, feel free to email me at **michael.zollo@hotmail.com**

I would also like to invite you to join my private Facebook community for extra support and guidance. It's a place to ask questions, share your favourite Keto recipes and your results to inspire others and to get some inspiration along your own journey.

Facebook group - Keto conquer 101, learn to win the weight loss game

Instagram - effortless_weightloss

My other publications available on Amazon

The Keto Effect for Women

The Intermittent Fasting Impact for Women

Introduction

I want to thank you for choosing this book!

Chaffles seem to be the latest food craze these days. What are chaffles? They are cheese waffles! Instead of using regular or nut-based flours, cheese is used as the base to make these delicious waffles. All that you need is a waffle maker. The great thing about chaffles is that they are low-carb and high in fat. So, chaffles are naturally keto-friendly.

The ketogenic or the keto diet is a diet high in fat and low on carbs. When you limit or even remove carbs from your diet altogether, your body no longer depends on glucose to provide energy. Instead, it starts using the reserves of fat present within your body along with the fats from the food you consume to produce energy. These fats are converted into ketones, which are then processed to provide your body with the energy needed to function optimally. This process is known as ketosis. As long as you don't consume excess carbs, your body will be in ketosis.

One of the main benefits of the keto diet is fat loss and weight loss. If you want to shed any abdominal fat, then this is the best diet for you. Since your body keeps burning fat once in ketosis, you will notice an overall improvement in your energy levels too. Apart from this, the keto diet helps stabilize your blood sugar and cholesterol levels. A combination of all these factors reduces the risk of various cardiovascular diseases.

While following the keto diet, about 70% of your daily calorie requirement will be from fatty foods, 20 to 25% from proteins, and the rest from carbs. By consuming naturally fatty foods, your overall calorie intake reduces, in turn this helps maintain a calorie deficit, which promotes weight loss! You can gain all these benefits by following the keto diet.

A great thing about chaffles is that you can even freeze them. So, on the weekend, you can whip up a batch of chaffles and then place them in an airtight container and freeze them. They can last you for up to a month, or even more when you store them properly. It will come in handy, especially if you think you don't have the time to prepare chaffles daily. All that you need to do is reheat them by popping them in the microwave or by using an air fryer.

At times, the chaffles might end up sticking to the grill. It usually happens when the chaffle isn't cooked all the way through and you try to lift or remove the lid. When the dough isn't fully cooked, it tends to leave a sticky residue once the griddle is opened. It takes about 3 to 4 minutes to prepare a chaffle and ensure that you follow the cooking time given in the recipes in this book.

If you are looking for easy chaffle recipes, then this is the perfect book for you! Not only are these recipes quite easy to cook, but they are keto-friendly too. So, you can stick to your keto diet while enjoying delicious food.

There are plenty of savory and sweet chaffle recipes to choose from. Since these recipes are all low carb, they will help improve your metabolism, keep your body in ketosis, and enhance your body's fat-burning metabolism. You don't have to spend hours cooking keto-friendly meals. Just ensure that you have all the necessary ingredients in your pantry, and that's about it.

Points to Remember to Make Perfect Chaffles

- Read the manufacturer's instructions carefully as the instructions may vary with different manufactures.
- Plug in the waffle maker and preheat the waffle maker before pouring in the batter. Most recipes use a mini waffle maker.
- Grease the waffle maker with some oil after it is preheated. This step and the previous step are common for all the recipes unless specified otherwise, and thus will not be mentioned in every recipe.
- Add a tablespoon of almond flour (optional) for every egg used in the basic recipe as it will help make better, crispier chaffles (just a suggestion). Also, using only egg whites makes crisp chaffles.
- All the ingredients should be at room temperature unless specified otherwise.
- Scatter a little cheese, preferably mozzarella cheese (apart from the cheese mentioned in the recipe) on the waffle maker initially. The cheese should cover the bottom of the waffle maker. Pour the batter over the cheese layer. Sprinkle some more cheese over the batter. This also helps in making crisp chaffles.
- Having patience is important. Do not keep opening the waffle maker every few minutes to check. It will delay the cooking.
- Once the chaffles are made, it is a great idea to brush them with butter.

Follow the instructions of the manufacturer for cleaning the waffle maker and the recipes mentioned below for preparing and cooking and you will be a master chaffle maker.

All nutritional info is based on the entire volume of recipe not per serve)

Chapter 1: Basic Chaffle Recipes

Basic Keto Chaffle with Egg and Mozzarella

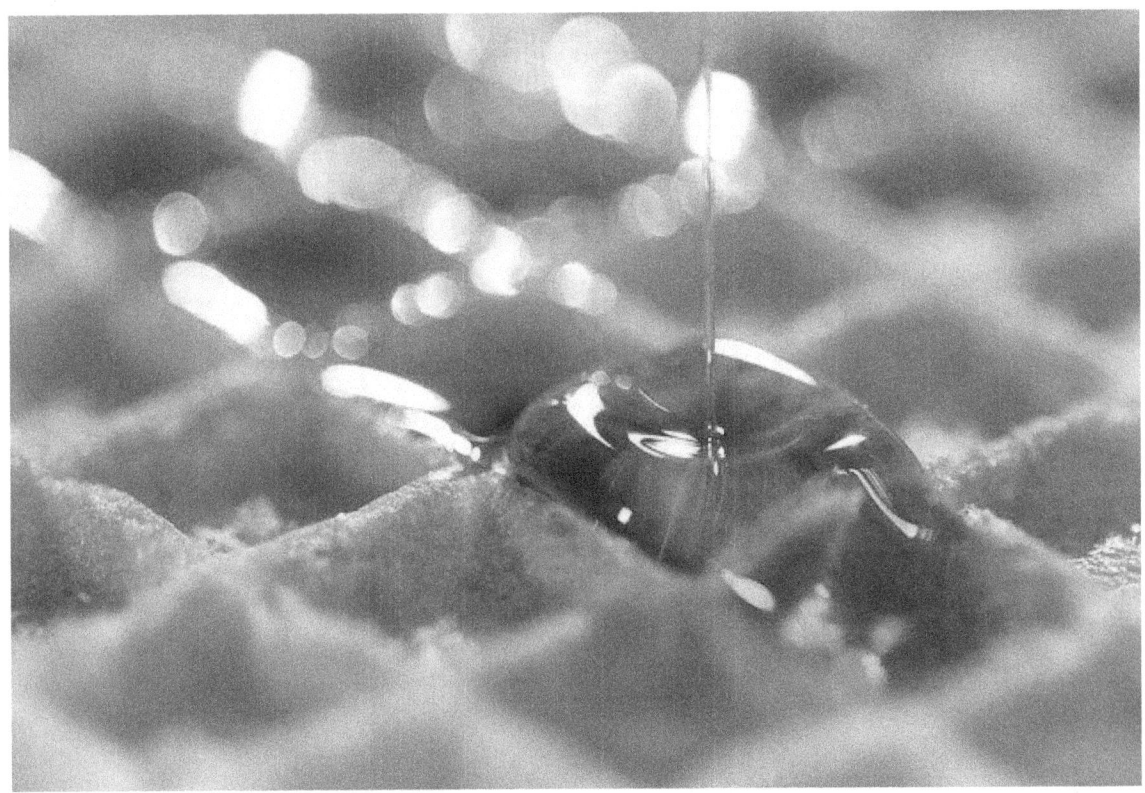

Makes: 4 waffles **Protein 33g Carb 4g Fat28g**

Ingredients:

- 1 cup finely shredded mozzarella cheese
- 2 large eggs

To serve:

- Keto-friendly toppings of your choice
- Melted butter, to brush

Directions:

1. Add eggs into a bowl and beat with a fork. Stir in the mozzarella.
2. Pour ¼ of the batter into the mini waffle maker. Set the timer for 2 to 3 minutes. Close the waffle maker.
3. When the timer goes off, check the chaffle. Cook for a couple of minutes more if required. Take out the chaffle and set aside on a plate. Let it sit for a couple of minutes.
4. Repeat steps 3 and 4 to make the remaining chaffles.
5. Brush with some melted butter. Serve with keto-friendly toppings of your choice.

Basic Keto Chaffle with Egg, Mozzarella and Almond Flour

Makes: 4 chaffles **Protein 46g Carbs 11g Fat 64g**

Ingredients:

- 1 cup finely shredded cheddar cheese
- 2 large eggs
- 4 tablespoons almond flour

To serve:

- Keto-friendly toppings of your choice
- Melted butter, to brush

Directions:

1. Add eggs into a bowl and beat with a fork. Stir in cheddar cheese and almond flour.
2. Pour ¼ of the batter into the mini waffle maker. Set the timer for 2 to 3 minutes. Close the waffle maker.
3. When the timer goes off, check the chaffle. Cook for a couple of minutes more if required. Take out the chaffle and set aside on a plate. Let it sit for a couple of minutes.
4. Repeat steps 2 and 3 to make the remaining chaffles.
5. Brush with some melted butter. Serve with keto-friendly toppings of your choice.

White Bread Keto Chaffle

Makes: 4 chaffles **Protein 21g Carbs 11g Fat 53g**

Ingredients:

- 2 eggs
- 2 tablespoons keto-friendly mayonnaise
- 2 teaspoons water
- 6 tablespoons almond flour
- ½ teaspoon baking powder

Directions:

1. Add eggs into a bowl and whisk with a fork. Whisk in rest of the ingredients.
2. Whisk in mayonnaise, almond flour, water and baking powder.
3. Pour ¼ of the batter into the mini waffle maker. Set the timer for 3 to 5 minutes. Close the waffle maker.
4. When the timer goes off, check the chaffle. Cook for a couple of minutes more if required. Take out the chaffle and set aside on a plate. Let it sit for a couple of minutes.
5. Repeat steps 3 and 4 to make the remaining chaffles.
6. Use instead of bread for sandwiches, with fillings of your choice.

Rye "Bread" Chaffle

Makes: 4 chaffles **Protein 82g Carbs 16g Fat 93g**

Ingredients:

- 2 cups shredded Swiss cheese
- 4 teaspoons caraway seeds
- ¼ teaspoon salt
- 4 eggs
- 1 teaspoon baking powder

Directions:

1. Add eggs into a bowl and whisk with a fork. Whisk in rest of the ingredients.
2. Pour ¼ of the batter into the mini waffle maker. Set the timer for 3 to 5 minutes. Close the waffle maker.
3. When the timer goes off, check the chaffle. Cook for a couple of minutes more if required. Take out the chaffle and set aside on a plate. Let it sit for a couple of minutes.
4. Repeat steps 2 and 3 to make the remaining chaffles.
5. Use instead of bread for sandwiches, with fillings of your choice.

Vegan Keto Chaffle

Makes: 4 chaffles **Protein 10g Carbs 37g Net Carbs 21g Fat 26g**

Ingredients:

- 2 tablespoons flaxseed meal
- ½ cup shredded low carb vegan cheese
- 2 tablespoons low carb vegan cream cheese, softened
- 5 tablespoons water
- 4 tablespoons coconut flour
- A pinch salt

Directions:

1. To make flax egg: Add flaxseed meal and water in a bowl and whisk it well. Keep it aside for 10 to 15 minutes.
2. Add rest of the ingredients into the bowl of flax eggs and whisk well.
3. Pour ¼ of the batter into the mini waffle maker. Set the timer for 4 to 5 minutes. Close the waffle maker.
4. When the timer goes off, check the chaffle. Cook for a couple of minutes more if required. Take out the chaffle and set aside on a plate. Let it sit for a couple of minutes.
5. Repeat steps 3 and 4 to make the remaining chaffles.

Chapter 2: Breakfast Sweet Chaffle Recipes

Chocolate Chip Chaffle with Whipped Cream

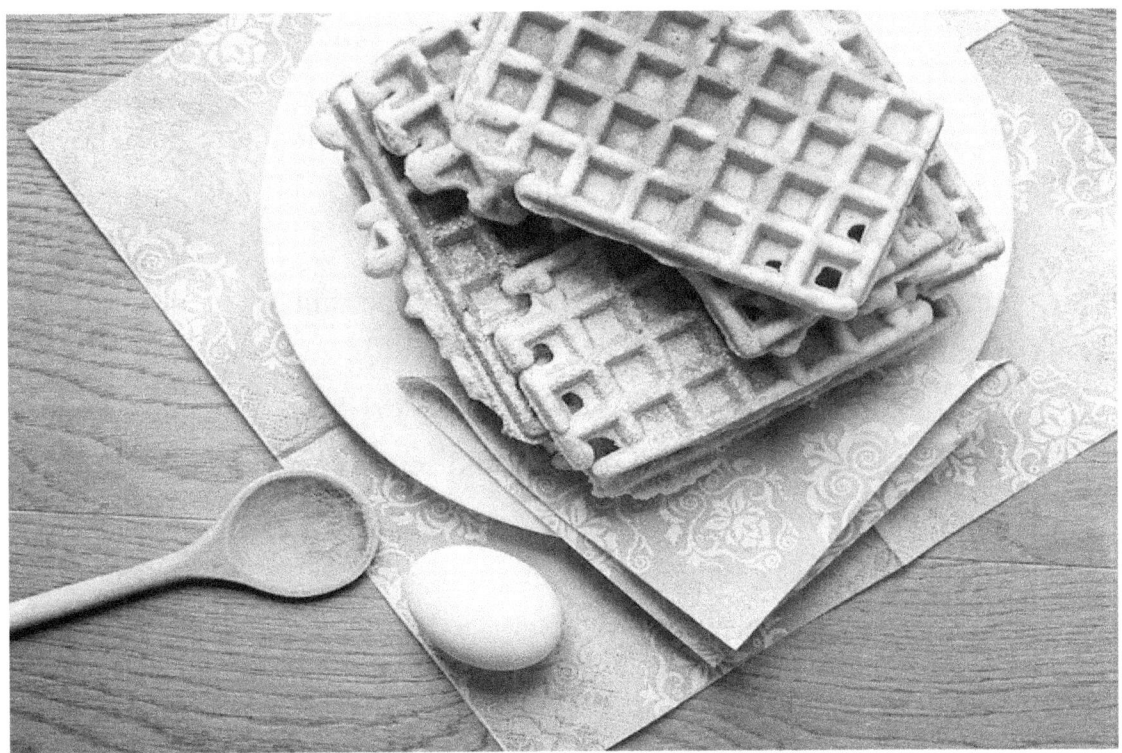

Makes: 4 chaffles **Protein 45g Carb 14g Net carb 10g Fat 52g** (whipped cream not counted for)

Ingredients:

For chaffles:

- 1 cup shredded mozzarella cheese
- 2 eggs
- 1 tablespoon granulated swerve

- 2 tablespoons almond flour
- ½ teaspoon ground cinnamon
- ¼ cup sugar-free chocolate chips

To serve:

- Whipped cream
- Powdered swerve or erythritol

Directions:

1. Add eggs, almond flour, swerve, mozzarella and cinnamon into a bowl and stir until well combined. Whisk well.
2. Add chocolate chips and stir.
3. Pour ¼ batter in the mini waffle maker. Set the timer for 4 minutes. Close the waffle maker.
4. When the timer goes off, check the chaffle. Cook for a couple of minutes more if required. Take out the chaffle and set aside on a plate. Let it sit for a couple of minutes.
5. Repeat steps 3 and 4 to make the remaining chaffles.
6. Sprinkle powdered swerve on top. Serve with whipped cream.

Cream Cheese Chaffles

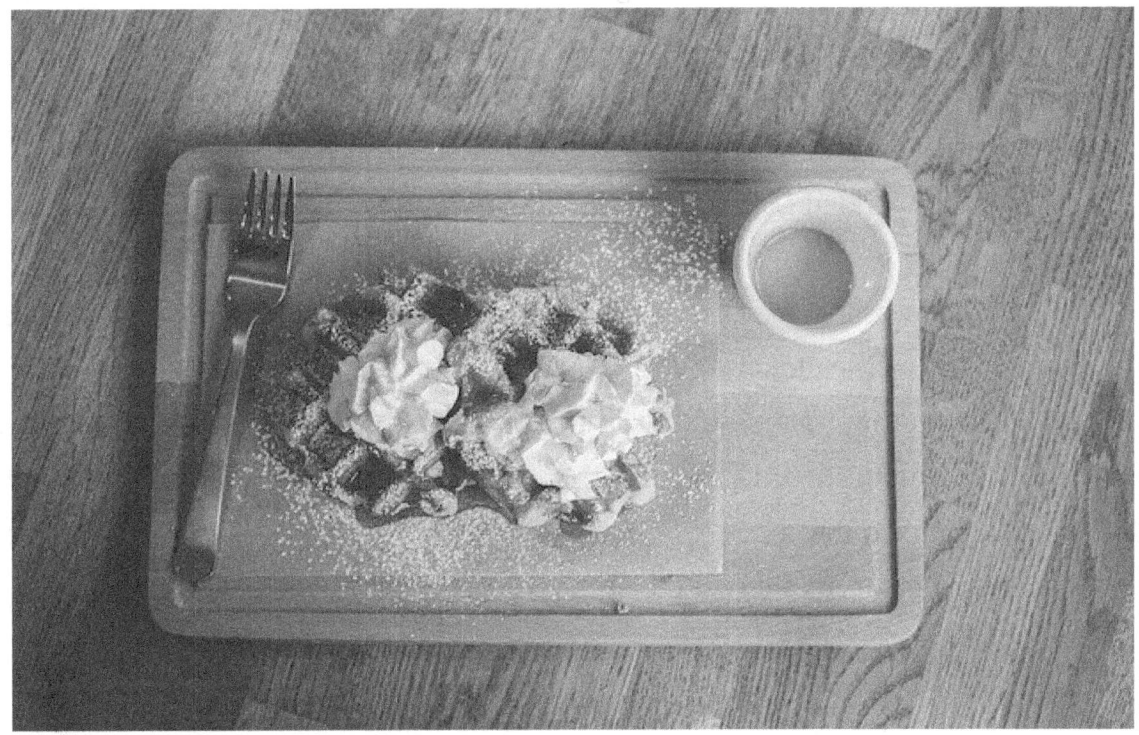

Makes: 4 chaffles **Protein 34g Carbs 34g Net carb 19g Fat 96g**

Ingredients:

- 4 eggs
- 3 tablespoons butter
- 4 ounces cream cheese
- ¼ teaspoon maple extract
- ½ teaspoon vanilla extract
- 2 tablespoons coconut flour
- 1 tablespoon erythritol
- 2 tablespoons oat fiber
- 1 ½ teaspoons baking powder
- 2 tablespoons almond milk

Directions:

1. Place 3 of the egg whites into a mixing bowl and the yolks into a blender along with the rest of the eggs, cream cheese, butter, vanilla and maple extract and blend until well combined.
2. Add all the dry ingredients and blend until smooth.
3. Whip the whites and beat until frothy.
4. Pour the blended batter into the bowl of whites. Fold gently. Do not over mix.
5. Pour ¼ of batter into the mini waffle maker. Set the timer for 4 minutes. Close the waffle maker.
6. When the timer goes off, check the chaffle. Cook for a couple of minutes more if required. Take out the chaffle and set aside on a plate. Let it stay for a couple of minutes.
7. Repeat steps 4, 5 and 6 to make the remaining chaffles.

Chocolate Chaffle

Makes: 4 chaffles **Protein 18g Carbs 11g Net carb 7g Fat 64g** (using butter not coconut oil)

Ingredients:

- 1 teaspoon baking powder
- ½ cup almond flour
- 3 tablespoon swerve or erythritol
- 2 tablespoons cacao powder or unsweetened cocoa powder
- 2 large eggs
- 1 teaspoon vanilla extract (optional)
- 4 tablespoons butter or coconut oil, melted

Directions:

1. Add all the wet ingredients into a bowl and whisk well.
2. Mix the dry ingredients into the bowl of wet ingredients. Stir until well combined.
3. Pour ½ the batter into the mini waffle maker. Set the timer for 4 minutes. Close the waffle maker.
4. When the timer goes off, check the chaffle. Cook for a couple of minutes more if required. Take out the chaffle and set aside on a plate. Allow it to sit for a couple of minutes.
5. Repeat steps 3 and 4 to make the remaining chaffles.

Banana Chaffle

Makes: 4 chaffles **Protein 42g Carb 11g Fat 44g**

Ingredients:

- 2 eggs
- 2 tablespoons sugar-free cheesecake pudding mix (optional)
- 2 tablespoons cream cheese, softened, at room temperature
- 2 tablespoons Monk fruit confectioners
- ½ teaspoon banana extract
- ½ teaspoon vanilla extract
- 1 cup shredded mozzarella cheese

To serve: Optional

- 2 tablespoons chopped pecans
- Sugar-free caramel sauce, to drizzle

Directions:

1. Whisk eggs in a bowl with a fork. Add the remaining ingredients and beat well.
2. Pour ¼ batter in the mini waffle maker. Set the timer for 4 minutes. Close the waffle maker.
3. When the timer goes off, check the chaffle. Cook for a couple of minutes more if required. Take out the chaffle and set aside on a plate. Let it sit for a couple of minutes.
4. Repeat steps 2 and 3 to make the remaining chaffles.
5. Drizzle caramel sauce on top if using. Sprinkle pecans and serve.

Chapter 3: Savory Breakfast Chaffle Recipes

Avocado Toast

Makes: 4 chaffles **Protein 54g Carb 20g Net carb 10g Fat 79g**

Ingredients:

For chaffle:

- 1 cup finely shredded mozzarella cheese
- 2 large eggs
- 2 teaspoons baking powder
- 2 tablespoons almond flour

For avocado topping:

- 1 avocado, peeled, pitted, mashed
- 2 teaspoons lemon juice
- Pepper to taste
- Salt to taste
- 1/8 teaspoon crushed red pepper
- 1 tablespoon olive oil
- 2 teaspoons butter, melted
- ½ cup feta cheese

Directions:

1. To make chaffles: Whisk eggs in a bowl with a fork. Add the remaining ingredients and beat well.
2. Pour ¼ of batter into the mini waffle maker. Set the timer for 4 minutes. Close the waffle maker.

3. When the timer goes off, check the chaffle. Cook for a couple of minutes more if required. Take out the chaffle and set aside on a plate. Let it sit for a couple of minutes.
4. Repeat steps 2 and 3 to make the remaining chaffles.
5. Place chaffles on a plate and brush with melted butter.
6. Meanwhile, add avocado, olive oil, lemon juice, salt, pepper and crushed red pepper and mix well.
7. Spread the avocado mixture on the chaffles. Sprinkle feta cheese on top and serve.

Scrambled Egg Chaffle

Makes: 4 chaffles **Protein 52g Carb 14g Net carb 8g Fat 110g**

Ingredients:

For chaffle:

- 2 eggs
- 2 tablespoons mayonnaise
- 2 teaspoons water
- 6 tablespoons almond flour
- ½ teaspoon baking powder

For scrambled eggs:

- 4 large free range eggs
- 3-4 tablespoons butter
- ¾ cup single cream or full cream milk
- Salt to taste
- Pepper to taste

Directions:

1. To make chaffles: Add eggs into a bowl and whisk with a fork. Whisk in rest of the ingredients.
2. Whisk in mayonnaise, almond flour, water and baking powder.
3. Pour ¼ of the batter into the mini waffle maker. Set the timer for 3 to 5 minutes. Close the waffle maker.
4. When the timer goes off, check the chaffle. Cook for a couple of minutes more if you want crisp chaffles. Take out the chaffle and set aside on a plate. Allow it to sit for a couple of minutes.

5. Repeat steps 3 and 4 to make the remaining chaffles.
6. To make scrambled eggs: Crack eggs into a bowl. Add cream or milk, pepper and salt and whisk lightly until well combined.
7. Place a nonstick pan over medium heat. Add butter. When butter melts, add the egg mixture. Do not stir for 20 seconds.
8. Using a wooden spoon, stir lightly. Lift and fold the egg over from the bottom of the pan.
9. Do not stir for another 10 seconds. Lift and fold the egg over from the bottom of the pan.
10. Repeat the previous step until the eggs are cooked soft overall but also runny at different spots. Turn off the heat.
11. Stir lightly.
12. Top chaffles with scrambled eggs and serve.

Keto Cornbread Chaffle

Makes: 4 **Protein 41g Carb 21g Net carb 17g Fat 46g**

Ingredients:

- 2 large eggs
- 10 to 12 slices jalapeños, fresh or pickled
- ½ teaspoon corn extract
- 1 cup shredded cheddar cheese
- 1/8 teaspoon salt
- 2 teaspoons Frank's red hot sauce

Directions:

1. Add eggs into a bowl and whisk with a fork. Whisk in the mozzarella, jalapeños, salt, corn extract and hot sauce.
2. Pour ¼ of the batter into the mini waffle maker. Set the timer for 3 to 5 minutes. Close the waffle maker.
3. When the timer goes off, check the chaffle. Cook for a couple of minutes more if required. Take out the chaffle and set aside on a plate. Let it sit for a couple of minutes.
4. Repeat steps 3 and 4 to make the remaining chaffles.

Garlic Parmesan Chaffles

Makes: 4 **Protein 52g Carb 4g Fat 42g** (Not including toppings)

Ingredients:

- 1 cup shredded mozzarella cheese
- ½ cup grated Parmesan cheese
- ½ teaspoon garlic powder
- 2 large eggs
- 2 teaspoons Italian seasoning

To serve:

- Olive oil
- Chopped fresh herbs of your choice
- Grated Parmesan cheese

Directions:

1. Beat eggs with a fork. Add garlic powder and Italian seasoning and whisk well.
2. Stir in the mozzarella and Parmesan cheese.
3. Pour ¼ of the batter into the mini waffle maker. Set the timer for 3 to 5 minutes. Close the waffle maker.
4. When the timer goes off, check the chaffle. Cook for a couple of minutes more if required. Take out the chaffle and set aside on a plate. Let it sit for a couple of minutes.
5. Repeat steps 3 and 4 to make the remaining chaffles.
6. To serve: Drizzle oil on top. Sprinkle herbs and Parmesan on top and serve.

Bacon, Lettuce and Tomato Breakfast Sandwich

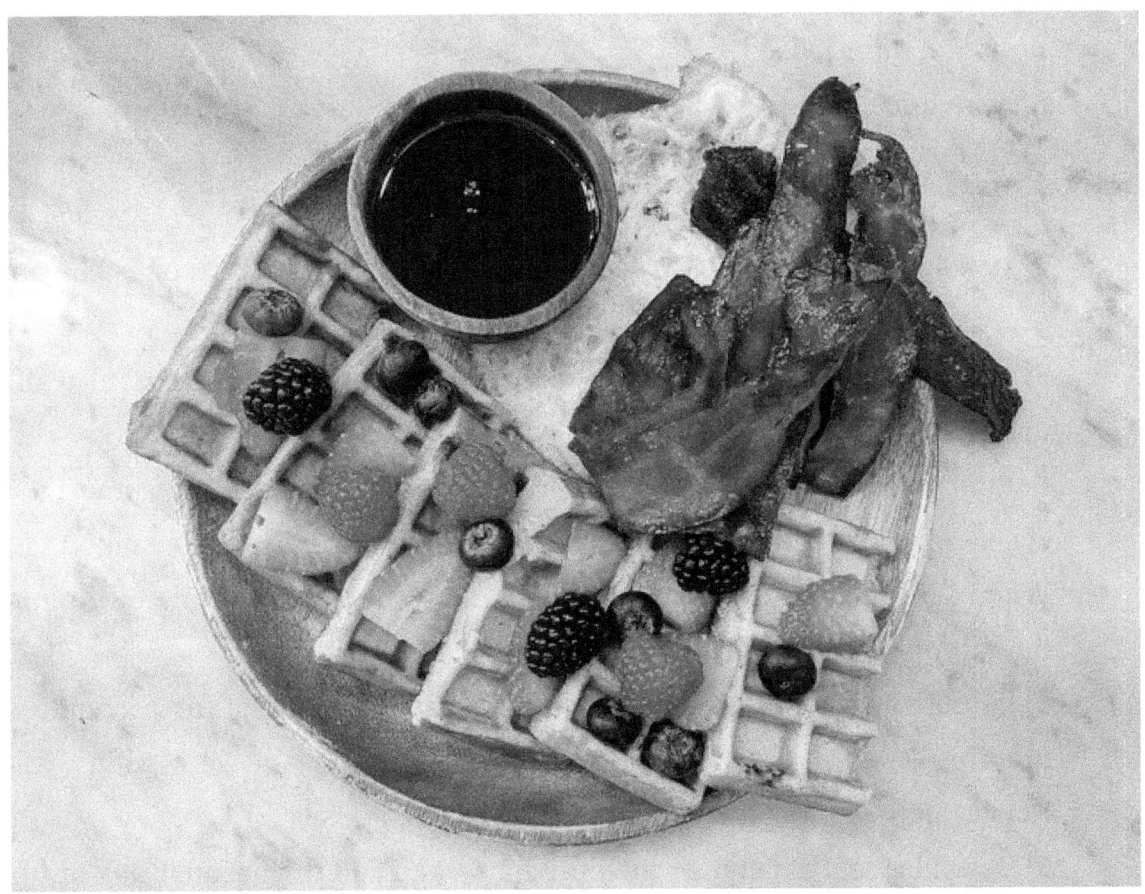

Makes: 2 sandwiches

Ingredients:

For chaffle: **Protein 45g Carb 7g Fat 48g** (allowing for 2 pieces of bacon)

- 1 cup shredded mozzarella cheese, plus extra
- 2 tablespoons sliced green onion
- 2 large eggs
- 1 teaspoon Italian seasoning
- Salt to taste (optional)

<u>For filling:</u>

- Bacon, as required
- 2 tablespoons mayonnaise
- 1 tomato, thinly sliced
- A few lettuce leaves

Directions:

1. Whisk eggs with a fork. Stir in the Italian seasoning, salt, mozzarella and green onion.
2. Sprinkle some extra mozzarella cheese on the bottom of the mini waffle maker.
3. Pour ¼ of the batter into the mini waffle maker. Sprinkle some more cheese on top. Set the timer for 3 to 5 minutes. Close the waffle maker.
4. When the timer goes off, check the chaffle. Cook for a couple of minutes more if required.
5. Take out the chaffle and set aside on a plate. Let it sit for a couple of minutes.
6. Repeat steps 2 and 5 to make the remaining chaffles.
7. Meanwhile, heat a pan over medium flame and add the bacon. Cook until it browns. Remove and set aside on paper towels. Turn off the heat.
8. Place 2 chaffles on a serving plate. Spread a tablespoon of mayonnaise on each.
9. Place bacon, lettuce and tomato slices over the chaffles. Cover with the remaining 2 chaffles. Cut into desired shape and serve.

Chapter 4: Lunch Chaffle Recipes

Bruschetta Chaffle

Makes: 4 chaffles **Protein 70g Carb10g Net carb 8g Fat 84g**

Ingredients:

- 1 cup shredded mozzarella cheese
- 2 large eggs
- 1 teaspoon Italian seasoning
- 2/3 cup grated Parmesan cheese
- ½ teaspoon garlic powder
- ½ teaspoon baking powder (optional)

For topping:

- 8 cherry tomatoes, chopped
- Extra-virgin olive oil to drizzle
- 1/8 teaspoon salt
- 1 teaspoon finely chopped basil
- ½ teaspoon balsamic vinegar
- 1 clove garlic, peeled, minced
- Red pepper flakes

Directions:

1. Beat eggs with a fork. Add garlic powder and Italian seasoning and whisk well.
2. Stir in the mozzarella and Parmesan cheese.
3. Pour ¼ of the batter into the mini waffle maker. Set the timer for 3 to 5 minutes. Close the waffle maker.

4. When the timer goes off, check the chaffle. Cook for a couple of minutes more if it is not crisp. Take out the chaffle and set aside on a plate. Let it sit for a couple of minutes.
5. Repeat steps 3 and 4 to make the remaining chaffles.
6. To make bruschetta topping: Add all the ingredients for bruschetta topping except oil into a bowl and toss well.

Spread the topping over the chaffles. Drizzle oil on top and serve.

Italian Chaffle Sandwich

Makes: 2 sandwiches **Protein 64g Carb 5 Fat 52g** (not counting toppings)

Ingredients:

- ½ cup grated Parmesan cheese
- 1 cup shredded mozzarella cheese
- 2 large eggs
- ½ teaspoon garlic powder
- 2 teaspoons Italian seasoning

For sandwich filling:

- 4 tablespoons chopped ham
- Salami slices, as required
- 2 tablespoons sliced olives
- Lettuce leaves
- Salt and pepper to taste
- Marinara sauce (keto-friendly) to drizzle
- Cheese slices

Directions:

1. Whisk eggs in a bowl with a fork. Stir in mozzarella, Italian seasoning, Parmesan cheese and garlic powder.
2. Pour ¼ of the batter into the mini waffle maker. Set the timer for 3 to 5 minutes. Close the waffle maker.
3. When the timer goes off, check the chaffle. Cook for a couple of minutes more if required. Take out the chaffle and set aside on a plate. Let it sit for a couple of minutes.
4. Repeat steps 3 and 4 to make the remaining chaffles.
5. Top with lettuce leaves, ham, salami, cheese and olives. Drizzle some marinara sauce on top. Cover with the remaining chaffles. Cut into desired shape and serve.

Reuben Chandwich

Makes: 2 sandwiches **Protein 82g Carb 14g Net carb 11g Fat 85g**

Ingredients:

For chaffle:

- 2 cups shredded Swiss cheese
- 4 teaspoons caraway seeds
- ¼ teaspoon salt
- 4 eggs
- 1 teaspoon baking powder

For filling:

- 4 tablespoons keto-friendly Russian dressing
- 2 ounces Swiss cheese
- 2 ounces corned beef or pastrami
- ½ cup sauerkraut

Directions:

1. Add eggs into a bowl and whisk with a fork. Whisk in rest of the ingredients.
2. Pour ¼ of batter into the mini waffle maker. Set the timer for 3 to 5 minutes. Close the waffle maker.
3. When the timer goes off, check the chaffle. Cook for a couple of minutes more if required to make crisp chaffles. Take out the chaffle and set aside on a plate. Allow it to sit for a couple of minutes.
4. Repeat steps 2 and 3 to make the remaining chaffles.
5. Spread a tablespoon of Russian dressing on each chaffle.

6. Place meat, sauerkraut and cheese on 2 of the chaffles. Close the sandwich with the remaining 2 chaffles, with the dressing side facing the filling.
7. Cut into desired shape and serve.

Ranch Slaw Sandwiches

Makes: 2 sandwiches **Protein 23g Carb 18g Net carb 11g Fat 54g**

Ingredients:

For chaffles:

- 2 eggs
- 2 tablespoons keto-friendly mayonnaise
- 2 teaspoons water
- 6 tablespoons almond flour
- ½ teaspoon baking powder

For ranch slaw:

- ¼ pound shredded coleslaw mix
- ½ tablespoon apple cider vinegar
- 1 to 2 tablespoons ranch dressing
- Salt to taste
- Pepper to taste

Directions:

1. Add the eggs into a bowl and whisk with a fork. Whisk in rest of the ingredients.
2. Whisk in mayonnaise, almond flour, water and baking powder.
3. Pour ¼ of batter into the mini waffle maker. Set the timer for 3 to 5 minutes. Close the waffle maker.
4. When the timer goes off, check the chaffle. Cook for a couple of minutes more if required. Take out the chaffle and set aside on a plate. Let it sit for a couple of minutes.

5. Repeat steps 3 and 4 to make the remaining chaffles. Cool completely.
6. To make ranch slaw: Add all the ingredients for ranch slaw into a bowl and mix it well. Refrigerate for 30 minutes.
7. Place 2 chaffles on a serving platter. Divide the coleslaw and spread over these chaffles. Close the sandwiches with the remaining chaffles.
8. Cut into desired shape and serve.

Pulled Pork Sandwich

Makes: 2 sandwiches **Protein 46g Carbs 18g Net carb 15g Fat 60g** (pulled pork not counted for)

Ingredients:

For chaffles:

- 1 cup finely shredded cheddar cheese
- 2 large eggs
- 4 tablespoons almond flour

For filling:

- Leftover pulled pork
- keto-friendly BBQ sauce, as required
- 2 tablespoons yellow mustard or as required

Directions:

1. Add eggs into a bowl and beat with a fork. Stir in cheddar cheese and almond flour.
2. Pour ¼ of the batter into the mini waffle maker. Set the timer for 2 to 3 minutes. Close the waffle maker.
3. When the timer goes off, check the chaffle. Cook for a couple of minutes more if required. Take out the chaffle and set aside on a plate. Let it sit for a couple of minutes.
4. Repeat steps 2 and 3 to make the remaining chaffles.
5. To make filling: Add pork and BBQ sauce into a pan and mix well. Place the pan over medium heat. Heat thoroughly.
6. Spread ½ tablespoon mustard on each chaffle. Place pulled pork mixture

on 2 of the chaffles. Cover with the remaining chaffles, with the mustard side facing down.

7. Cut into desired shape and serve.

Tuna Salad Chaffle Sandwich

Makes: 1 sandwich **Protein 27g Carb 9g Net carb 7g Fat 34g**

Ingredients:

For chaffle:

- ½ cup finely shredded mozzarella or cheddar cheese
- 1 large egg
- 2 tablespoons superfine, blanched almond flour
- ¼ teaspoon + 1/8 teaspoon baking powder
- ¼ teaspoon garlic powder

For tuna salad filling:

- 2 tablespoons canned tuna, drained
- 2 tablespoons sliced celery
- 2 tablespoons mashed avocado
- 1 small clove garlic, minced
- 1 tablespoon mayonnaise
- Lemon juice to taste
- Salt to taste
- Pepper to taste
- 1 tablespoon diced cucumber
- 1 tablespoon minced onion

Directions:

1. To make chaffle: Whisk eggs, almond flour, baking powder and garlic powder in a bowl. Stir in mozzarella cheese.
2. Spoon ½ the batter into the mini waffle maker. Set the timer for about 10

minutes. Close the waffle maker.

3. When the timer goes off, check the chaffle. Cook for a couple of minutes more if required. Take out the chaffle and set aside on a plate. Allow it to sit for a couple of minutes.
4. Repeat steps 2 and 3 to make the remaining chaffle.
5. To make filling: Add all the ingredients for tuna salad into a bowl and mix well.
6. Place a chaffle on a serving platter. Spread filling over it. Cover with the remaining chaffle. Cut into the desired shape and serve.

Chapter 5: Dinner Chaffle Recipes

Corndog Chaffle

Makes: 8 to 10 corndog chaffles **Protein 69g Carbs 14g Net carb 12g Fat 34g**

Ingredients:

- 4 eggs
- 2 tablespoons almond flour
- ½ teaspoon salt or to taste
- 2 cups Mexican blend cheese
- 1 teaspoon cornbread extract
- 8 to 10 hotdogs with its sticks

To serve:

- Mustard
- Mayonnaise
- keto-friendly ketchup, etc.

Directions:

1. Whisk eggs in a bowl. Add the remaining ingredients and whisk well.
2. Grease a corndog waffle maker with some cooking spray and let it preheat.
3. Pour the batter into the corndog waffle maker. Fill up to half. Place hot dogs with its stick in each cavity and press it into the cavity slightly.
4. Smear some batter on top of the hot dogs. Close the waffle maker.
5. Set the timer for 4 minutes or until golden brown.
6. Using a pair of tongs, remove the hotdog chaffles. Let it cool for 5 minutes.
7. Serve with any of the suggested serving options.

Keto Sausage Ball Chaffle

Makes: 8 to 10 chaffles **Protein 414g Carb 138g Net carb 105g Fat 340g**

Ingredients:

- 2 pounds bulk Italian sausage
- 4 teaspoons baking powder
- ½ cup grated Parmesan cheese
- 2 cups almond flour
- 2 cups shredded sharp cheddar cheese
- 2 large eggs or flax eggs (2 tablespoons flaxseeds mixed with 6 tablespoons water)

<u>To serve:</u> Use any (optional)

- Sour cream
- keto-friendly marinara sauce
- keto-friendly ranch dressing
- Sugar-free maple syrup

Directions:

1. Add eggs, cheddar cheese, Parmesan cheese, baking powder, Italian sausage and almond flour into a bowl. Mix well using your hands.
2. Spread 3 tablespoons of the batter into the regular waffle maker. Set the timer for 3 to 4 minutes. Close the waffle maker.
3. When the timer goes off, flip sides and cook for 2 minutes. Cook for longer if you want crisp chaffles. Take out the chaffle and set aside on a plate. Let it sit for a couple of minutes.
4. Repeat steps 2 and 3 to make the remaining chaffles.

Chicken Sandwich

Makes: 2 sandwiches **Protein 186g Carb 58g Net carb 24g Fat 228g**

Ingredients:

For chaffle bun:

- 2 cups finely shredded mozzarella cheese
- 2 eggs
- ½ teaspoon butter extract
- 6 to 10 drops stevia glycerite

For chicken filling:

- 2 chicken breasts
- 4 tablespoons powdered Parmesan cheese
- 2 teaspoons ground flaxseeds
- 4 tablespoons butter, melted
- ½ cup dill pickle juice
- 4 tablespoons ground pork rinds
- Salt to taste
- Pepper to taste

Directions:

- For chaffle buns: Add all the ingredients except mozzarella into a bowl. Whisk well. Stir in the mozzarella.
- Pour ¼ of the batter into the mini waffle maker. Set the timer for 2 to 3 minutes. Close the waffle maker.
- When the timer goes off, check the chaffle. Cook for a couple of minutes more if required. Take out the chaffle bun and set aside on a plate. Let it sit

for a couple of minutes.
- Repeat steps 2 and 3 to make the remaining chaffle buns.
- To make filling: Place the chicken breasts on your countertop. Pound with a meat mallet until it is ½ inch thick. Cut each into 2 halves.
- Place the chicken in a large Ziploc bag. Pour pickle juice over the chicken. Seal the bag. Turn the bag around a few times so that the chicken is well coated with the juice. Let it marinate for 1 to 8 hours.
- Remove from the refrigerator 30 minutes before cooking. Discard the marinade and remove the chicken from the bag.
- Place flaxseeds, pork rinds, Parmesan cheese, salt and pepper in a shallow bowl and stir.
- First brush butter generously over the chicken. Next dredge chicken in the pork rind mixture.
- Cook in a preheated air fryer or an oven at 400°F for about 8 to 10 minutes or until cooked through.
- Place 2 chaffle buns on a serving platter. Place one piece of chicken on each chaffle bun. Cover with the remaining chaffles and serve.

BBQ Chicken Chaffle

Makes: 4 chaffles **Protein 73g Carb 27g Net carb 25g Fat 54g**

Ingredients:

For chaffle:

- 2/3 cup cooked, diced chicken
- 2 tablespoons keto-friendly BBQ sauce, plus extra to serve
- 2 tablespoons almond flour
- 1 cup shredded cheddar cheese
- 2 eggs

Directions:

1. Add eggs, BBQ sauce and almond flour into a bowl and whisk it until well combined.
2. Add chicken and cheddar cheese and mix well.
3. Pour ¼ of batter in the mini waffle maker. Set the timer for about 4 minutes. Close the waffle maker.
4. When the timer goes off, check the chaffle. Cook for a couple of minutes more if required.
5. Take out the chaffle and set aside on a plate. Allow it to sit for a couple of minutes.
6. Repeat steps 4 and 6 to make the remaining chaffle.
7. Serve with BBQ sauce.

Keto Taco Chaffle

Makes: 4 chaffles **Protein 66g Carb 8g Net carb 6g Fat 53g** (not counting fillings)

Ingredients:

- ½ teaspoon Italian seasoning
- 2 large eggs
- ½ teaspoon salt
- 1 cup shredded mozzarella cheese
- 2 tablespoons almond flour
- ¼ teaspoon baking soda

For taco filling:

- ½ teaspoon keto-friendly taco seasoning
- ¼ pound ground beef or turkey

For toppings:

- Shredded lettuce
- Cheese
- Cherry tomatoes, halved
- Sour cream
- Any other keto-friendly toppings of your choice

Directions:

1. To make chaffles: Add eggs, salt, Italian seasoning, baking soda and almond flour into a bowl and whisk well.
2. Stir in the mozzarella.
3. Spoon ¼ of the batter into the waffle maker. Set the timer for 2 to 3

minutes. Close the waffle maker.
4. When the timer goes off, check the chaffle. Cook for a couple of minutes more if required.
5. Take out the chaffle and place on top of an inverted bowl (smaller than the chaffle). Let it remain in this position for some time until it cools. This will be the taco shell.
6. Repeat steps 3 and 5 to make the remaining chaffle.
7. To make taco meat: Add meat into a pan. Place the pan over medium heat and cook until it turns light brown. Add the taco seasoning and cook until brown, then turn off the heat.

Place taco meat in the taco shells and serve with suggested toppings.

Chaffle Pizza

Makes: 4 chaffles **Protein 43g Carbs 8g Net carbs 6g Fat 41g** (not counting toppings)

Ingredients:

- 2 eggs
- ½ teaspoon dried basil or to taste
- 1 cup shredded mozzarella cheese
- 1 teaspoon baking powder
- ½ teaspoon garlic powder
- 2 tablespoons almond flour

For topping:

- 4 tablespoons shredded mozzarella cheese
- 2 mushrooms, sliced
- 2 black olives, thinly sliced
- 4 tablespoons keto-friendly pasta sauce or pizza sauce
- Any other toppings of your choice

Directions:

1. For chaffles: Add eggs, dried basil, almond flour, baking powder and garlic powder and into a bowl and whisk together.
2. Add mozzarella cheese and whisk well.
3. Pour ¼ of the batter into the waffle maker. Set the timer for about 3 to 4 minutes. Close the waffle maker.
4. When the timer goes off, check the chaffle. Cook for a couple of minutes more if required.
5. Repeat steps 4 and 6 to make the remaining chaffles.
6. Place chaffles on a baking sheet. Spread a tablespoon of pasta sauce on top

of each of the chaffles. Sprinkle a tablespoon of cheese on each. Place mushrooms, olives and any other keto-friendly toppings of your choice.

7. Bake in a preheated oven at 375° F for 5 minutes.

Chapter 6: Vegan Chaffle Recipes

Savory Chaffle

Makes: 4 chaffles **Protein 37g Carb 34g Net carb 13g Fat 69g**

Ingredients:

- 2 tablespoons coconut cream
- 12 tablespoons almond flour
- 2 teaspoons chives
- ½ teaspoon onion powder
- Salt to taste
- 2 flax eggs (2 tablespoons flaxseeds mixed with 5 tablespoons water and set aside for 10 to 12 minutes)
- ½ teaspoon xanthan gum
- ¼ teaspoon garlic powder
- Pepper to taste

Directions:

1. Mix all the ingredients in a bowl and whisk into a thick batter.
2. Pour ¼ of batter to the mini waffle maker. Set the timer for about 3 to 4 minutes. Close the waffle maker.
3. When the timer goes off, check the chaffle. Cook for a couple of minutes more if required.
4. Repeat steps 2 and 3 to make the remaining chaffles.

Churros Chaffle

Makes: 4 chaffles **Protein 37g Carb 36g Net carb 13g Fat 69g**

Ingredients:

- 2 tablespoons coconut cream
- 12 tablespoons almond flour
- 1 teaspoon ground cinnamon
- 2 flax eggs (2 tablespoons flaxseeds mixed with 5 tablespoons water and set aside for 10 to 12 minutes)
- ½ teaspoon xanthan gum
- 4 tablespoons Sukrin Gold

Directions:

1. Add all ingredients in a bowl and whisk into a thick batter.
2. Pour ¼ of batter into the mini waffle maker. Set the timer for about 3 to 4 minutes. Close the waffle maker.
3. When the timer goes off, check the chaffle. Cook for a couple of minutes more if required.
4. Repeat steps 2 and 3 to make the remaining chaffles.

Chocolate Chaffle

Makes: 4 chaffles **Protein 47g Carb 57g Net carb 25g Fat 90g**

Ingredients:

- 2 tablespoons coconut cream
- 12 tablespoons almond flour
- 2 tablespoons cocoa powder
- 2 flax eggs (2 tablespoons flaxseeds mixed with 5 tablespoons water and set aside for 10 to 12 minutes)
- ½ teaspoon xanthan gum
- 4 tablespoons Sukrin Gold
- 4 tablespoons keto friendly, vegan chocolate chips

Directions:

1. Add all ingredients in a bowl and whisk into a thick batter.
2. Pour ¼ of the batter into the mini waffle maker. Set the timer for about 3 to 4 minutes. Close the waffle maker.
3. When the timer goes off, check the chaffle. Cook for a couple of minutes more if required.
4. Repeat steps 2 and 3 to make the remaining chaffles.

Vanilla Belgian Chaffle

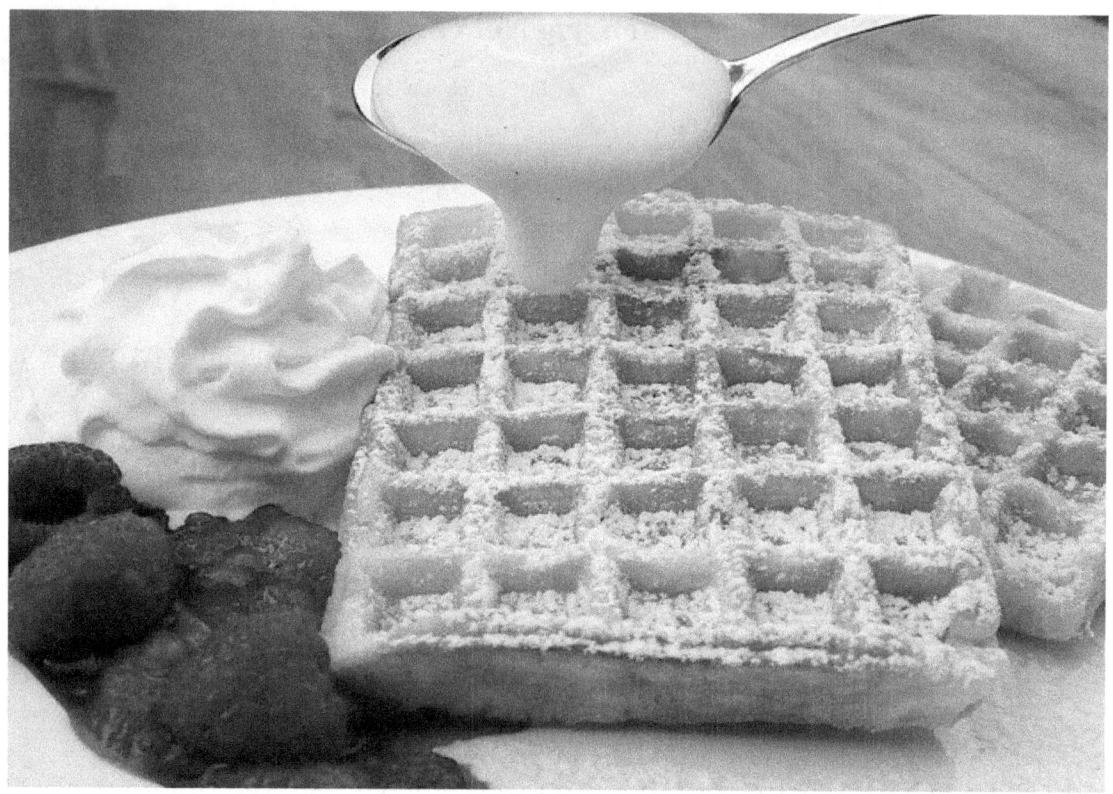

Makes: 4 chaffles **Protein 25g Carb 46g Net carb 22g Fat 45g**

Ingredients:

- ½ cup shredded low carb vegan cheese
- 2 tablespoons low carb vegan cream cheese, softened
- 5 tablespoons water
- 4 tablespoons coconut flour
- A pinch salt
- 2 flax eggs (2 tablespoons flaxseeds mixed with 5 tablespoons water and set aside for 10 to 12 minutes)
- 4 tablespoons Sukrin Gold
- 2 teaspoons vanilla extract

Directions:

1. Add all ingredients in a bowl and whisk into a thick batter.
2. Pour ¼ of the batter into the mini waffle maker. Set the timer for about 3 to 4 minutes. Close the waffle maker.
3. When the timer goes off, check the chaffle. Cook for a couple of minutes more if required.
4. Repeat steps 2 and 3 to make the remaining chaffles.

Pumpkin Chaffle

Makes: 4 chaffles **Protein 38g Carb 40g Net carb 17g Fat 69g**

Ingredients:

- 2 tablespoons coconut cream
- 12 tablespoons almond flour
- 4 tablespoons pumpkin puree
- 2 flax eggs (2 tablespoons flaxseeds mixed with 5 tablespoons water and set aside for 10 to 12 minutes)
- ½ teaspoon xanthan gum
- 4 tablespoons Sukrin Gold
- 2 teaspoons pumpkin pie spice

Directions:

1. Add all ingredients in a bowl and whisk into a thick batter.
2. Pour ¼ of the batter into the mini waffle maker. Set the timer for about 3 to 4 minutes. Close the waffle maker.
3. When the timer goes off, check the chaffle. Cook for a couple of minutes more if required.
4. Repeat steps 2 and 3 to make the remaining chaffles.

Chapter 7: Snack Chaffle Recipes

Chaffle Churro

Makes: 16 sticks **Protein 40g Carbs 10g Fat 34g**

Ingredients:

- 2 eggs
- 4 tablespoons swerve brown sweetener
- 1 cup shredded mozzarella cheese
- 1 teaspoon ground cinnamon

Directions:

1. Beat eggs with a fork. Stir in the mozzarella.
2. Pour ¼ of the batter into the mini waffle maker. Set the timer for 3 to 4 minutes or until golden brown. Close the waffle maker.
3. Take out the chaffle and place on a plate. Cut into 4 slices while it is hot.
4. Place sweetener and cinnamon on a plate and mix well. Dredge the sticks in this mixture immediately and place on a serving platter
5. Repeat steps 2 and 4 to make the remaining chaffles.

Breadsticks

Makes: 16 sticks **Protein 65g Carb 10g Net carb 9g Fat 52g**

Ingredients:

- ½ cup grated Parmesan cheese
- 1 cup shredded mozzarella cheese
- 2 large eggs
- ½ teaspoon onion powder
- 1 tablespoon minced herbs of your choice

To serve:

- Grated Parmesan cheese
- Minced fresh herbs
- Marinara sauce
- Olive oil

Directions:

1. Beat together eggs and onion powder with a fork. Stir in the herbs, mozzarella and Parmesan cheese.
2. Spoon ¼ of the batter into the mini waffle maker. Set the timer for 2 to 3 minutes. Close the waffle maker.
3. When the timer goes off, check the chaffle. Cook for a couple of minutes more if required.
4. Take out the chaffle and set aside on a plate. Cut into 4 strips.
5. Repeat steps 2 and 4 to make the remaining chaffles.
6. Place on a baking sheet.
7. Place the bread sticks on a serving platter. Sprinkle Parmesan cheese. Bake for a few minutes in the oven until cheese melts.
8. Garnish with herbs. Drizzle olive oil on top and serve with marinara sauce.

Pickle Flavored Chaffle Sticks

Makes: 16 sticks **Protein 42g Carb 26g Net carb 25g Fat 48g**

Ingredients:

- 1 cup shredded mozzarella cheese
- 2 large eggs
- 2 tablespoons pickle juice
- ½ cup pork panko
- 12 to 15 thin pickle slices, pat dry with paper towels

For dip:

- 2 tablespoons ranch dressing
- Hot sauce

Directions:

1. Beat eggs and pickle juice with a fork. Stir in the mozzarella and pork panko.
2. Pour ¼ of the batter into the mini waffle maker. Scatter 3 to 4 pickle slices. Set the timer for 4 minutes. Close the waffle maker.
3. When the timer goes off, check the chaffle. Cook for a couple of minutes more if required.
4. Take out the chaffle and place on a plate. Cut into 4 slices.
5. Repeat steps 2 and 4 to make the remaining chaffles.

Garlic Breadsticks

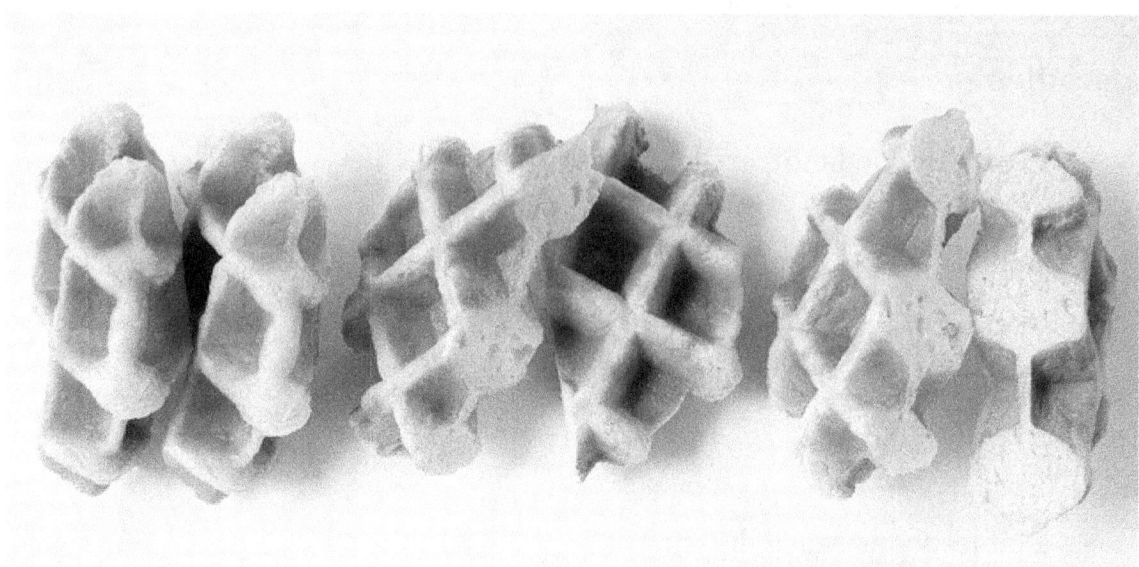

Makes: 16 breadsticks **Protein 89g Carb 13g Net carb 10g Fat 128g**

Ingredients:

- 1 cup shredded mozzarella cheese
- 2 eggs
- 4 tablespoons almond flour
- Salt to taste
- 2/3 cup grated Parmesan cheese
- 2 large cloves garlic, minced or 1 teaspoon garlic powder

For topping:

1. 4 tablespoons unsalted butter, softened
2. ½ cup grated mozzarella cheese
3. 1 teaspoon garlic powder

Directions:

1. Beat eggs with a fork. Stir in mozzarella, garlic, almond flour, Parmesan cheese and salt.
2. Spoon ¼ of batter into the mini waffle maker. Set the timer for 5 minutes. Close the waffle maker.
3. Take out the chaffle and place on a plate. Cut into 4 strips.
4. Repeat steps 3 and 4 to make the remaining chaffles.
5. Place the sticks on a baking sheet in a single layer.
6. Add butter and garlic powder into a bowl and stir. Spread this mixture over the sticks.
7. Sprinkle cheese on top.
8. Preheat the oven in broil mode. Broil it for two minutes. Serve.

Savory Cauliflower Chaffle Sticks

Makes: 16 sticks **Protein 92g Carb 16g Net carb 11g Fat 70g**

Ingredients:

- 2 cups grated cauliflower
- ½ teaspoon salt or to taste
- ½ teaspoon pepper or to taste
- 1 cup shredded mozzarella cheese or Mexican cheese blend
- 2 large eggs
- 1 teaspoon Italian seasoning
- 1 cup grated Parmesan cheese, plus extra for the waffle maker
- ½ teaspoon garlic powder
- ½ teaspoon baking powder (optional)

Directions:

1. Add all the ingredients in a blender and blend well. Pour into a bowl.
2. Sprinkle 2 tablespoons Parmesan cheese on the bottom of the mini waffle maker.
3. Pour ¼ of batter into the mini waffle maker. Set the timer for 3 to 5 minutes. Close the waffle maker.
4. When the timer goes off, check the chaffle. Cook for a couple of minutes more if required.
5. Take out the chaffle and set aside on a plate. Cut into 4 strips.
6. Repeat steps 2, 3, 4 and 5 to make the remaining chaffles.

Chapter 8: Dessert Chaffle Recipes

Blueberry Chaffle Muffin

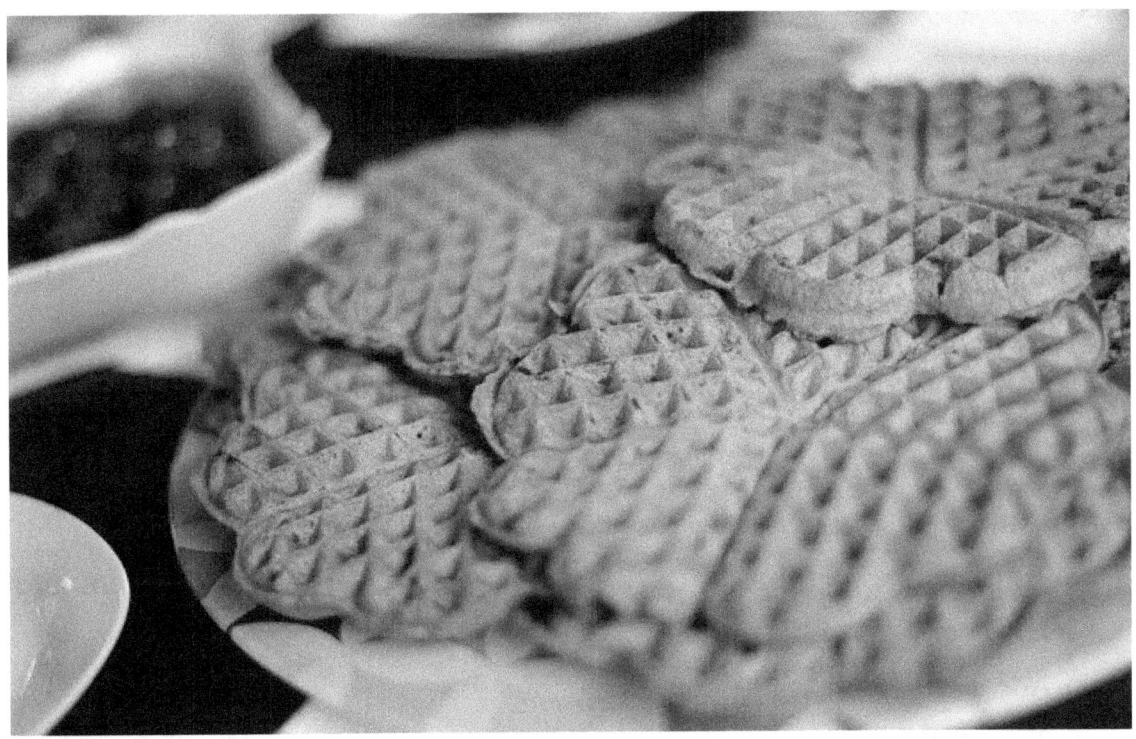

Makes: 24 chaffle muffins **Protein 132g Carb 67g Net carb 45g Fat 134g**

Ingredients:

- 6 eggs
- ½ cup coconut flour
- 2 tablespoons swerve sweetener
- 3 cups finely shredded mozzarella cheese
- 2 teaspoons baking powder
- ½ cup blueberries
- ½ teaspoon vanilla extract

For frosting (optional):

- 2 tablespoons cream cheese, softened
- 4 tablespoons powdered erythritol or swerve
- 6 tablespoons whipping cream

Directions:

1. Beat egg with a fork. Add vanilla and whisk well. Stir in mozzarella cheese.
2. Add coconut flour, baking powder and swerve into a bowl and stir until well combined. Add into the bowl of eggs. Mix well.
3. Add blueberries and fold gently.
4. Grease 2 muffin pans of 12 counts each.
5. Divide the batter among the muffin cups.
6. Bake in a preheated oven at 350°F for 30 minutes or until done.
7. Remove the pans from the oven and allow it to cool.
8. Run a knife around the edges of the muffins and invert onto a plate.
9. To make frosting (if using): Add cream cheese and whipping cream into a bowl and beat until smooth.
10. Add swerve and beat until well combined.
11. Transfer the frosting into a piping bag and pipe the frosting over the muffins and serve.

Nutty Bread Pudding

Makes: 3 servings **Protein 42g Carb 27g Net carb 23g Fat 134g**

Ingredients:

For chaffles:

- 1 tablespoon butter, melted, cooled
- 1 large egg
- 1 ounce cream cheese
- 2 tablespoons almond flour
- 2 tablespoons swerve confectioners
- 1 tablespoon coconut flour
- ½ teaspoon baking powder
- ½ teaspoon vanilla extract
- ½ teaspoon ground cinnamon
- A pinch Himalayan pink salt

Other ingredients for pudding:

- 1 egg, beaten
- ¼ cup swerve or sukrin gold
- 2 tablespoons heavy whipping cream
- 1 teaspoon vanilla extract
- ½ teaspoon ground cinnamon
- 1 teaspoon banana extract
- ¼ teaspoon ground nutmeg
- 1 ¼ cups lukewarm milk of your choice

For topping:

- ½ cup chopped nuts
- 1 tablespoon sukrin gold
- 3 tablespoons butter, melted

To serve:

- Whipped cream

Directions:

1. To make chaffle: Add all the wet ingredients into a bowl and whisk well.
2. Add the dry ingredients and combine well.
3. Pour ½ the batter into the mini waffle maker. Set the timer for 4 minutes. Close the waffle maker.
4. When the timer goes off, check the chaffle. Cook for a couple of minutes more if required. Take out the chaffle and set aside on a plate. Allow it to sit for a couple of minutes.
5. Repeat steps 3 and 4 to make the remaining chaffles.
6. When the chaffles have cooled completely, chop into 1-inch squares.
7. Place chaffle pieces in a baking dish or casserole dish.
8. Add all the other ingredients for pudding into a bowl and whisk well. Pour into the casserole dish over the chaffles. Stir to coat.
9. To make topping: Add butter, sukrin gold and nuts into a bowl and mix well. Scatter on top of the casserole.
10. Bake in a preheated oven at 350°F for about 30 minutes.
11. Remove from the oven and allow it to cool before serving.

Ice Cream Chaffle Sandwich

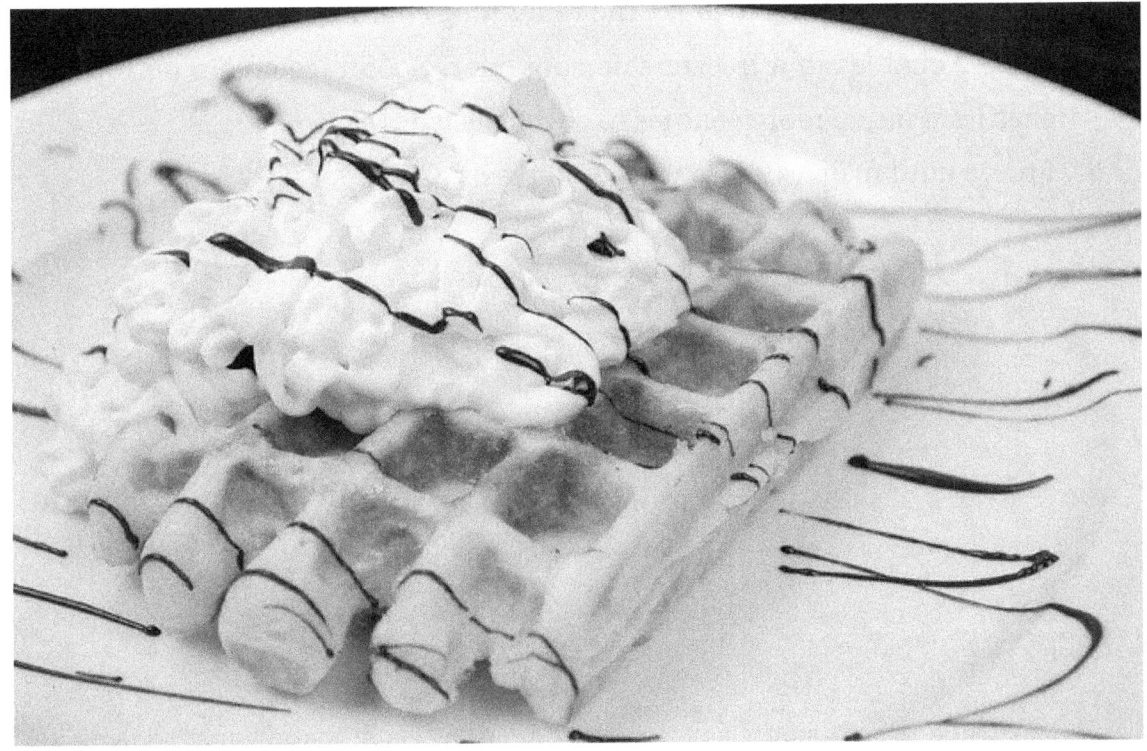

Makes: 6 to 8 servings **Protein 24g Carb 47g Net carb 35g Fat 26g**

Ingredients:

- 4 tablespoons cocoa
- 2 eggs
- 2 tablespoons heavy whipping cream
- 4 tablespoons monk fruit confectioners
- ½ teaspoon baking powder
- Keto ice cream of your choice

Directions:

1. Add all the ingredients except ice cream into a bowl and whisk well.
2. Pour ¼ of the batter into the mini waffle maker. Set the timer for about 3

to 4 minutes. Close the waffle maker.
3. When the timer goes off, check the chaffle. Cook for a couple of minutes more if required.
4. Repeat steps 2 and 3 to make the remaining chaffles.
5. Place 2 chaffles in a freezer safe container. Spoon ice cream on top of the chaffles. Place 2 more chaffles to cover the ice cream.
6. Freeze until firm. Cut into wedges and serve.

Strawberry Shortcake Bowls

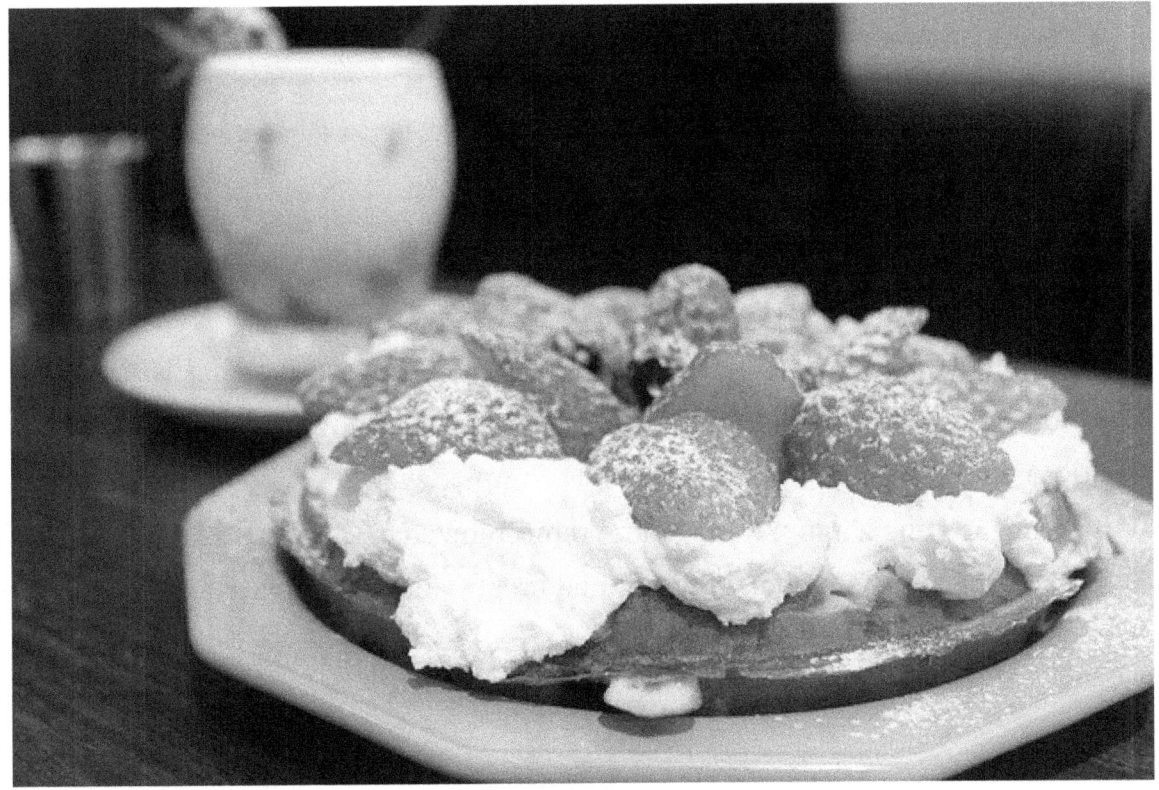

Makes: 2 servings **Protein 20g Carb 11g Net carb 7g Fat 19g** (Not counting what you service it with)

Ingredients:

- 2 egg whites
- 1 egg
- ¼ cup almond flour
- ½ teaspoon ground cinnamon or to taste
- 1 teaspoon stevia or to taste
- ½ teaspoon baking powder
- 4 strawberries, chopped

To serve:

- Low carb whipped cream
- Few strawberries, sliced
- Confectioners' swerve

Directions:

1. Add all ingredients in a bowl and whisk well.
2. Pour ¼ of the batter into the mini waffle maker. Set the timer for about 3 to 4 minutes. Close the waffle maker.
3. When the timer goes off, check the chaffle. Remove the chaffle and place on an inverted bowl. It will take the shape of the bowl. Let it remain in this position for some time until it cools completely.
4. Repeat steps 2 and 3 to make the remaining chaffles.
5. Mix together strawberries, whipped cream and swerve into a bowl. Fill the chaffle bowls with this mixture and serve.

"Apple" Fritter Chaffles

Makes: 2-3 chaffles **Protein 15g Carb 19g Net carb 11g Fat 37g**

Ingredients:

For "apple" fritter filling:

- 1 cup diced jicama
- 2 tablespoons butter
- A pinch ground nutmeg
- ¼ teaspoon vanilla
- 10 drops apple extract
- 2 ½ tablespoons swerve sweetener blend
- ½ teaspoon ground cinnamon
- A pinch ground cloves

For chaffles:

- 1 egg
- ½ teaspoon coconut flour
- ½ tablespoon almond flour
- ¼ teaspoon baking powder
- ¼ cup grated mozzarella cheese

For glaze:

- ½ tablespoon butter
- 1 ½ tablespoons powdered swerve
- 1 teaspoon heavy cream
- 1/8 teaspoon vanilla extract

Directions:

1. Place a skillet over medium-low heat. Add butter. When butter melts, add jicama and swerve and stir.
2. Lower the heat to low heat and cover with a lid. Cook until tender.
3. Turn off the heat. Add rest of the ingredients for filling and mix well.
4. To make chaffles: Add egg, flours and baking powder into a bowl and whisk well.
5. Add jicama mixture and mix well.
6. Sprinkle a tablespoon of cheese on the preheated mini waffle maker.
7. Spread 2 heaping tablespoons of the batter into the waffle maker.
8. Sprinkle another tablespoon of cheese over the batter.
9. Set the timer for 2 to 3 minutes. Close the waffle maker.
10. When the timer goes off, check the chaffle. Cook for a couple of minutes more if required. Take out the chaffle and set aside on a plate. Let it sit for a couple of minutes.
11. Repeat steps 6 – 10 and make the remaining chaffles.
12. To make glaze: Add butter into a small saucepan. Place the saucepan over medium heat. When butter melts, add cream and swerve and cook until thick. Turn off the heat.
13. Add vanilla and stir. Spoon over the chaffles. Let the icing cool before serving.

Sugar Cookie

Makes: 4 cookies

Ingredients:

For cookies:

- 2 tablespoons butter, melted
- 2 egg yolks
- ¼ teaspoon cake batter extract
- ¼ teaspoon baking powder
- 2 tablespoons swerve
- ¼ teaspoon vanilla extract
- 6 tablespoons almond flour

For icing:

- 2 tablespoons confectioners
- 2-4 teaspoons water
- ½ teaspoon vanilla
- To sprinkle:
- 2 tablespoons granular sweetener
- 1-2 drops food coloring

Directions:

1. Whisk together all the ingredients for chaffle in a bowl. Let the batter sit for 5 minutes. Chill for 5 minutes.
2. Pour ¼ of the batter into the mini waffle maker. Set the timer for 4 minutes. Close the waffle maker.

3. When the timer goes off, check the chaffle. Cook for a couple of minutes more if required. Take out the chaffle and set aside on a plate. Let it sit for a couple of minutes.
4. Repeat steps 2 – 3 and make the remaining chaffles.
5. Whisk together all the ingredients for icing in a bowl. Spread over the chaffle. Scatter sprinkles on top and serve.

Conclusion

I want to thank you once again for choosing this book.

The chaffle is the latest keto creation, and it is something you will undoubtedly love. It makes for a great addition to your Sunday brunch too! A chaffle is a tasty snack or even a meal by itself! It is a keto-style waffle made of eggs and cheese while eliminating all carbs.

If you have been following the keto diet and were craving for some delicious waffles, then chaffles will certainly satiate this craving. You can do all this without worrying about compromising your diet. By following the keto diet, you can essentially attain your weight loss goals while eating delicious food!

It hardly takes any time to cook a chaffle, but be patient while it cooks. Resist the urge to open the waffle maker and peek at the chaffle while it cooks. If you do this, the chaffle will stick to the girdle! Whenever you are making a chaffle, don't overstuff it. If you do this, the batter will overflow, and you will need to clean the mess up. It is quite easy to clean the waffle iron. All that you need is a wet paper towel! To avoid the chaffle from sticking, ensure that the waffle iron is hot before adding all the ingredients. Start cooking these chaffles in batches and freeze them! When you store them in an airtight container, they can last you a couple of weeks. Cooking has never been this easy!

All the instructions given in this book are quite easy to follow and simple to cook. It hardly takes about 5 to 15 minutes to cook a delicious chaffle. Ensure that your pantry is stocked with all the keto-friendly ingredients you need; it becomes easier to cook. Now, all that's left for you to do is pick a recipe and start cooking. Once you make a chaffle, you will realize how easy cooking is! It barely takes any time to cook, and you don't have to worry about cleaning several pots and pans!

The key to attain your weight loss goal lies in your hands. So, what are you waiting for? Gather all the ingredients you need and start making delicious chaffles!

Don't forget

Go to www.vipketoreport.com to download your copy of the 7 keto foods you need to avoid for a successful diet plan

Also join my Facebook group at

keto conquer 101, learn to win the weight loss game

Follow me on Instagram at

effortless_weightloss

Thank you and all the best!

References

Pitre, U. (2019). Chaffles: The Best Keto Waffles You Need to Try ASAP!. Retrieved from https://twosleevers.com/chaffles-the-best-keto-waffle-recipes/

www.ingramcontent.com/pod-product-compliance
Lightning Source LLC
Chambersburg PA
CBHW060534010526
44107CB00059B/2638